Phyllis I. Dal

M000086457

Cranberry

The Cure for Common and Chronic Conditions

- **Urinary tract infections**
- **Eye disorders**
- **And others**

alive books

Vancouver
Canada

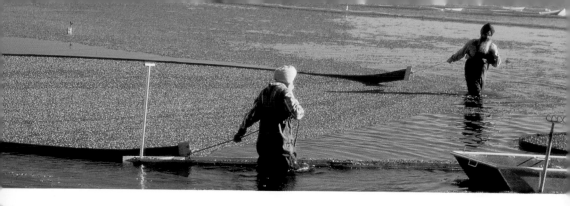

Contents

All About Cranberry

Note: Conversions in this book (from imperial to metric) are not exact. They have been rounded to the nearest measurement for convenience. Exact measurements are given in imperial. The recipes in this book are by no means to be taken as therapeutic. They simply promote the philosophy of both the author and *alive* books in relation to whole foods, health and nutrition, while incorporating the practical advice given by the author in the first section of the book.

Healthy Recipes

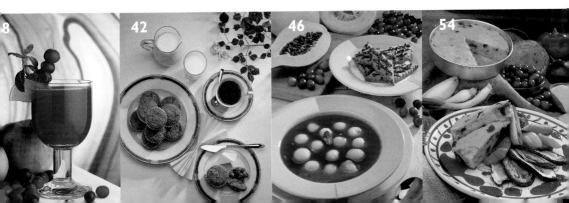

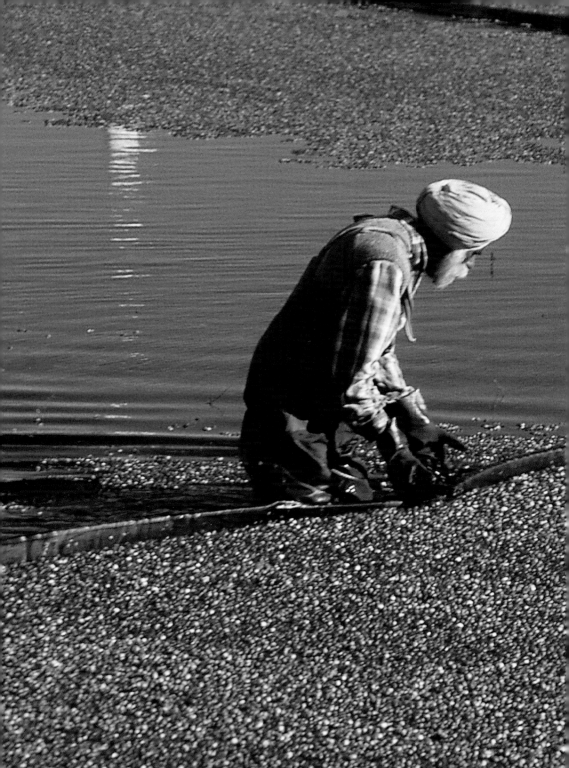

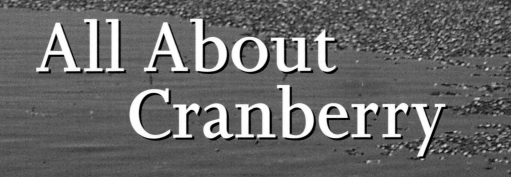

All About Cranberry

The cranberry is so effective in its healing that both Western medicine and the natural health field are recommending and relying on its benefits.

Introduction . . . .

The cranberry finally appears to be receiving the recognition it deserves for its healing powers. In fact, it is becoming as closely associated with bladder infections as vitamin C is with the common cold–and for good reason! However, the healing ability of this beautiful berry is nothing new. The mighty little cranberry has been treating and preventing ailments and disease for centuries.

Therapeutic applications of this natural remedy documented during the 17th century included the relief of blood disorders, stomach ailments, liver problems, vomiting, appetite loss, scurvy and cancer. In Eastern Europe cranberries were traditionally used to reduce fevers and treat cancer. Of course, in the United States in the 1820s, the Pilgrims were taught by the Native Americans to preserve cranberries. This led the Pilgrims to start the tradition of serving them as a delicacy with wild turkey at Thanksgiving.

I have my own fond memories concerning the cranberry. Growing up in the 1940s, I used to pick cranberries near my parents' farm in Manitoba. As the Pilgrims did, my mother would take the harvest of berries my father, sisters and I brought home and make them into jams and jellies–preserves to accompany a roasted turkey at Christmas time.

The cranberry, a relative of the blueberry, was traditionally used by Native Americans as both food and medicine.

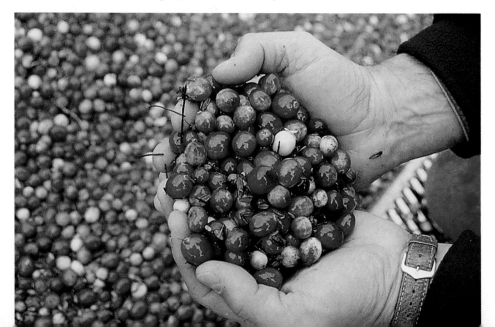

Years later the cranberry helped me regain my health and continues to help me maintain it. In 1988, adding to a history of health challenges, a terrible evening of tests and operations ended with a diagnosis of acute kidney failure. When leaving the hospital weeks later, my physician said I would require dialysis one to four times a month for the rest of my life.

Thankfully, with proper medical attention my kidneys began working slowly, but I still had high uric acid and creatine blood levels. My kidney condition and urinary tract infections are now under control. I am convinced that, along with changes to my diet and good medical care, it was my dedication to the cranberry that helped me return to health and to keep my kidney condition, and the urinary tract infections to which it made me susceptible, under control. My only relapse occurred when I stopped taking freeze-dried cranberry capsules for a ten-day period. Today, I am free of dialysis and have not seen my nephrologist (kidney specialist) in five years.

I was so impressed with the personal success I experienced with cranberry as a cure that, along with the help of my son, I devoted hundreds of hours to researching this amazing berry. I also shared my experience with as many people possible. I've received many letters relaying success stories.

One such letter was from a man who lived in the country but had moved to the city because he was told by physicians that he would require regular kidney dialysis within three months. He began taking cranberry capsules and one month later his kidney blood functions were within the normal range. He was able to keep off dialysis for an additional year.

The cranberry also provides hope for people who believe they must be on a regular dose of antibiotics, which cause a host of other health problems (see "Cranberry and the Urinary Tract Infection" section in this book), to prevent their bladder infections. Many letters also describe benefits in addition to relief of urinary tract infections, including great help with eye disorders.

The cranberry is so effective in its healing that both Western medicine and natural health circles alike are recommending and relying on its benefits. We have much to gain by learning about and using the benefits of the cranberry. Let's do so now!

The cranberry is becoming as closely associated with bladder infections as vitamin C is with the common cold.

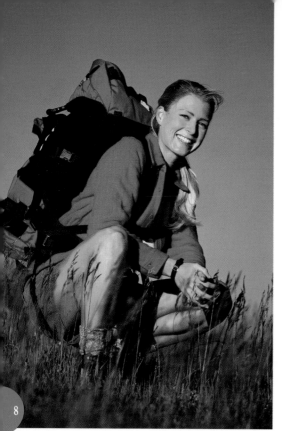

Cranberry and the Urinary Tract Infection · · · · · · · ·

The cranberry is best known for its ability to both prevent and treat urinary tract infections, which are most commonly known as bladder and kidney infections. To understand how the simple cranberry can cure these infections, we must first understand the basics of the urinary tract and the infections that occur there.

The Urinary Tract

The urinary tract consists of all the structures through which the urine passes, from the time it is formed until it leaves the body. Urinary tract infections can be found in one or all of these elements: the kidneys, ureters, urinary bladder, urethra and in the male prostate.

Cranberry is widely used today to prevent bladder infections.

Kidneys: The human kidney circulates more fluid than any other organ in the body. The kidneys (there are two of them) are located on either side of the spinal column, just below the diaphragm. These hard-working organs filter out and remove waste products from the blood, maintain a normal range of nutrients in the blood and regulate the acidbase (pH) balance in the body.

Ureters: These are the tubes that transport urine from the kidneys to the bladder.

Urinary bladder: The bladder acts as a holding tank for urine until it leaves the body through excretion.

Urethra: The urethra is the tube that transports urine from the bladder for excretion.

What Causes Urinary Tract Infections?

Bladder infections are caused by bacteria, which cause an inflammation of the bladder's inner lining. The bacteria *Escherichia coli*, which is beneficial to the lower bowels, is hazardous if it finds its way to the urinary organs; this is the most common cause of bladder infections. Females are more prone to urinary tract infections than are males because the female urethra is short, and situated close to the rectum, allowing bacteria to enter the bladder more easily.

Bladder infections may also be caused by being chilled–sitting on a cold surface or wearing damp clothing, for example. In men, bladder infections may be linked to prostate problems. Antibiotics (usually prescribed for these infections), birth control pills, stress and a poor diet all weaken the immune system and create a tendency for recurring infections.

Kidney infections can result from untreated bladder infections when bacteria invade the kidneys. Once again, getting a chill, especially in the lower back and pelvic area, increases a person's susceptibility to infection.

Symptoms of Urinary Tract Infections

- A burning sensation when urinating
- Frequent voiding or urination but only in small amounts
- Foul-smelling urine
- Cloudy urine
- Pain in lower abdomen
- Chills, fever
- Vomiting
- Lower-back pain whether you are moving about or not
- Edema (swelling), especially around the ankles, feet, hands and eyes
- Passing blood when urinating
- Difficulty urinating–this can happen in both sexes; in men, it could indicate an enlarged prostate
- Feeling the need to strain to begin urinating

How Cranberry Prevents and Cures . . . .

For centuries cranberries have been recommended and consumed for their beneficial effect on urinary tract infections. Researchers in Germany were studying the connections between cranberries and urinary tract infections as early as the 1840s. They found that people who ate cranberries had hippuric acid in their urine. By the turn of the century, researchers in the US were assuming that cranberries acidified urine, because of the hippuric acid results, and thereby prevented infection. However,

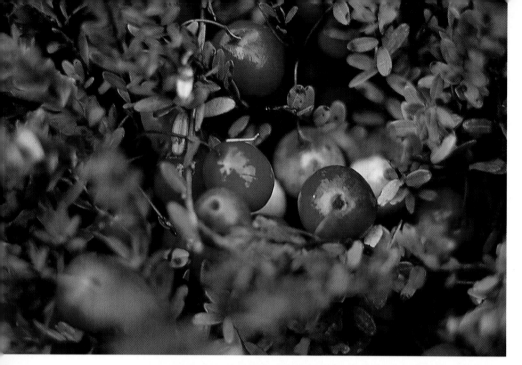

a strong belief in cranberries as a prevention method did not take hold because researchers failed to show that cranberries increased urine acidity enough to prevent infection.

Today, researchers are again studying the relationship between cranberries and a healthy urinary tract, but from a different angle. New research focuses on the cranberry's potential to keep bacteria from attaching to urinary tract walls.

New research focuses on the cranberry's potential to keep bacteria from attaching to urinary tract walls.

Some people have a natural substance (a mucoprotein), called *Tamm-Horsfall glycoprotein*, present in their urine. This substance has the ability to attach itself to the E. coli bacteria (which is responsible for about 85 percent of all urinary tract infections) and inhibit them from attaching to the bladder wall. People who have enough Tamm-Horsfall glycoprotein have much less chance of getting a urinary tract infection. In 1994, researchers at Weber State University in Utah discovered that cranberries contain a substance similar in activity to the Tamm-Horsfall glycoprotein.

I've had dozens of people write to me about their successes with cranberries for both preventing and treating urinary tract infections. One such letter was from a registered nurse in Manitoba, who said, "I recommended freeze-dried cranberry capsules to a friend with a history of kidney infections. While on these cranberry capsules there was no recurrent infection. However, when the capsules ran out a kidney infection developed." Another person swears that since taking cranberries therapeutically, he has been without a urinary tract infection for two years. He said, "Even my physician is surprised how much they've helped me."

Cranberry Content · · · · · · · · · · · · · · · ·

The wonderfully healing cranberry contains about 88 percent water. It is a good source of fiber, protein and vitamin A and is low in calories: 250 milliliters (1 cup) contains only 55 calories. Cranberries keep for up to eight weeks and freeze very well with no preparation. Fresh cranberries contain high amounts of vitamins, minerals, organic acids and various other phytonutrients (nutritious substances from plants).

Vitamins and Minerals in Cranberry

Vitamin Content

Vitamin A (beta-carotene)	Vitamin B_6 (pyridoxine)
Vitamin B_1 (thiamine)	Folacin (folic acid)
Vitamin B_2 (riboflavin)	Vitamin C (ascorbic acid)
Vitamin B_3 (niacin)	Vitamin E (alpha-tocopherol)
Vitamin B_5 (pantothenic acid)	

Mineral Content

Boron	Magnesium	Selenium
Calcium	Manganese	Sodium
Chromium	Molybdenum	Sulfur
Copper	Phosphorous	
Iron	Potassium	

Organic Acids

One of the distinguishing aspects of cranberry, particularly in comparison with other berries in the same family, is its high organic acid level, which is considered a phytonutrient of cranberry. The high organic acid level is the main reason it has a sour taste, and strong evidence indicates that the high organic acid level is related to its therapeutic value.

The benzoic acid in cranberries acts as a preservative and antifungal agent, keeping them fresh for a remarkably long time.

The main organic acids in cranberry—malic, quinic and citric acids—are all healthful. Malic acid, for example, helps guard against diarrhea and regulates digestion.

Phytonutrients

Cranberries have been found to contain a large variety of phytonutrients. Phytonutrients (also known as phytochemicals) are the biologically active substances in plants that give them

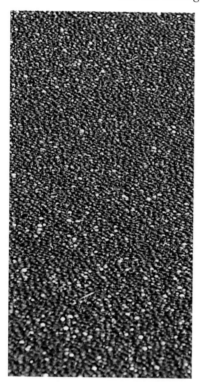

their color, flavor and their own natural resistance to disease.

Researchers have been working to isolate these phytonutrients, which are best known for the hope they provide in the prevention of cancer. There are literally thousands of phytonutrients to be discovered and more are being discovered each day.

The cranberry contains many of the recently discovered and well-known phyto-nutrients, such as:
- anthocyanins
- catechins
- chlorogenic acid
- eugenol
- lutein
- proanthocyanidins
- quercetin.

While manufacturers are producing and marketing phytonutrients individually, it is best to receive the full spectrum of phytonutrients and other benefits available from eating the real thing.

Quality Counts

The nutrient content of cranberries can vary greatly, depending on:
- the quality of the cranberry plant
- the quality of the soil in which they are grown
- season and climate
- harvesting conditions
- drying and storage conditions
- the manufacturing process

Contamination

Whether the cranberry is being used as food or for therapeutic use, it is important that it be as free from contamination as possible.

How are you storing your cranberry product? At one time many people stored their tablets and capsules in the bathroom. However, because of the heavy humidity in the bathroom from showering or bathing, it is best to keep them in a dry area.

Most foods contain minute amounts of heavy metals. As with any food, it is essential that the cranberries be grown on good-quality land, and that they be processed by a reputable manufacturer, to minimize heavy-metal contamination. Some of these heavy metals are cadmium, cobalt, lead and mercury. What level of heavy metals is safe? That depends on how much cranberry is being consumed. If it is going to be taken in therapeutic amounts, the manufacturer should guarantee a minimum of less than 10 parts per million total combined heavy metals and less than 3 parts per million lead.

Microbiological contamination may be an issue as well. To ensure that the product is safe, the manufacturer should perform quality control tests to make sure bacteria and mold levels are within the acceptable range. The product should be free of pathogenic bacteria (E. coli, Salmonella and Streptococci) as well. Pesticides can also be an issue. Manufacturers must be aware and act accordingly.

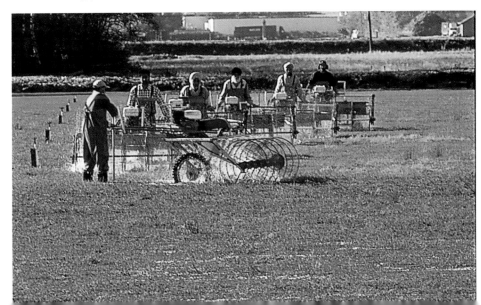

As with any product, to achieve successful results, cranberries must be high quality and produced by a reputable manufacturer.

Are you purchasing a quality product? Ask your retailer these questions:

- How much actual cranberry does the product contain?

- How much water and sweetener does it contain?

- What kind of sweetener does the product contain? If an artificial sweetener has been used, children should avoid the product.

- How has the cranberry been preserved?

- Has an artificial flavoring been used in place of real cranberries?

- How much of the product, whether juice, tablet or capsule, is required to receive therapeutic value?

- Has the product been made by a reliable manufacturer?

- Does the weight of the product correspond with the quality or quantity of therapeutic components in the juice, capsule or tablet?*

- How long will the product keep its therapeutic or nutritional potency before degrading?

- Has anything been added to the product to make it sell better? (If so, are you allergic to it?)

*Weight does not indicate potency. If the water level is low, the weight is low. Containing less water makes it a more concentrated product and gives it a longer shelf life. Keep in mind that all cellular reactions (such as mold growth) require water. Less water means fewer cellular reactions over time, and therefore better storage.

Cranberry Consumption · · · · · · · · · ·

Historically, cranberries have been used both as a food and for their therapeutic benefits. These benefits include, among many others, the prevention and treatment of urinary tract infections, prevention of scurvy, treatment of cancer, treatment of eye disorders, fever reduction and use as a poultice for a variety of conditions.

Cranberries are tasty and nutritious. The reason you decide to consume cranberries will dictate the form in which you choose to consume them. If your goal is to prevent or treat a condition, you certainly won't achieve the same results from eating sugar-sweetened cranberry sauce as you will from investing in unsweetened, pure cranberry juice or therapeutic freeze-dried cranberry capsules—or better yet, fresh, raw cranberries.

Fresh, Raw Cranberries

Eating fresh, raw cranberries is absolutely the most nutritious and healing way of consuming cranberries. Cranberries in this form will deliver the maximum therapeutic value. However, because of the cranberry's tart taste they are seldom eaten this way. They are also seasonal, and very few people have access to a cranberry farm. However, when available, and if you can acquire a taste for them, the whole-food form is very rewarding.

Composition of Cranberries		
	Cranberries, Raw (1 cup/113 grams)	Cranberry Sauce Sweetened, Canned or Cooked (1 cup/227 grams)
Food Energy (calories)	54	549
Protein (g)	0.5	0.3
Fat (g)	0.8	0.8
Total Carbohydrates (g)	12.8	142.4
Calcium (mg)	16	22
Phosphorus (mg)	12	19
Iron (mg)	0.7	0.8
Vitamin A (iu)	50	80
Vitamin B_1 Thiamine (mg)	0.03	0.06
Vitamin B_2 Riboflavin (mg)	0.02	0.06
Vitamin B_2 Complex	0.1	0.3
Vitamin C - Ascorbic Acid (mg)	13	5

Home Freezing

Freezing stops all cellular reactions in the cranberry, successfully preserving the product along with its nutritional value. Because of this, freezing is generally considered a better preservation method than canning. When thawing the berries, however, a small amount of the nutritional and therapeutic value may be lost. Cranberries should be frozen when they are at the peak of freshness. The only preparation required before freezing is that you wash the berries well.

Cooked Cranberry

In 1923, according to Blatherwick and Long in the *Journal of Biological Chemistry*, the acidity of the urine did not change significantly after a person ate cooked prunes. However, a person who ate 305 grams of cooked cranberries had his

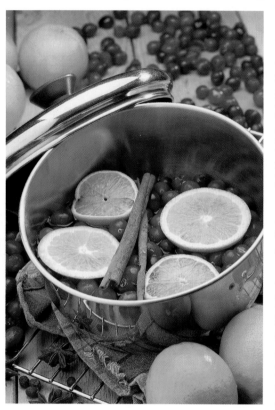

urinary pH level decreased from 6.4 to 5.3, with a subsequent increase in the excretion of total acids. It would appear that cooked cranberries do retain some of their nutritional value in comparison to other fruits; however, most people add sugar to cooked cranberries, which greatly lessens the nutritional value. Find a more nutritional substitute, such as honey, or go without a sweetener.

It just isn't Christmas or Thanksgiving without traditional cranberry sauce, but is the sauce nutritious? As a matter of fact, it is. As early as 1914, N.R. Blatherwick, in his writings for the *Archives of Internal Medicine*, showed the specific role of foods in relation to the composition of urine. Four people took part in a study about increasing urine acidity. It was found that all had increased urine acidity after eating 300-600 grams of cranberry sauce on a daily basis for a specific period. In 1923, Blatherwick and Long, in their studies of urinary acidity, showed that urine acidity was due mostly to the excretion of hippuric acid found after ingesting cranberries.

Natural, Unprocessed Cranberry Juice

Fresh-picked cranberries are approximately 88 percent water. The juice contains a wealth of vitamins, minerals and other nutrients. The major organic acids in the juice are malic, quinic and citric acids.

Cranberry Juice Cocktail

A cranberry juice cocktail usually is a mixture of cranberry juice and other liquids, such as apple juice and water. While many of the commercial cocktails contain very little cranberry juice, a cocktail is a tasty and beneficial way to enjoy cranberries.

As reported in the *New York State Journal of Medicine* in 1968, researchers Zinseer et al used cranberries as an acidifying agent in a nine-year study of fifty-three patients who were prone to kidney stones. Each patient consumed 1 quart of cranberry juice cocktail daily. At the end of the study, 32 percent of the patients with stones had no change, 60 percent improved and 8 percent worsened. The intervals between recurrences of infected stones were prolonged from twenty-one months to forty-four months for the individuals using the juice. Larger doses of undiluted cranberry juice were found to be even more effective in preventing urinary tract infections. Zinseer and colleagues noted the juice to be a simple and effective method of preventing and treating kidney infection.

Commercial Cranberry Drinks

Many cranberry drinks on the market contain only a very small amount of cranberry juice. Commercially bottled cranberry drinks with a reasonable shelf life must go through heat processing to sterilize them so that they can stay at room temperature without yeast, mold or bacteria build-up. The overwhelming majority of these products have been sweetened either with sugar, sugar substitute or another fruit juice. Quite often water is added to dilute the product. This decreases both the nutritional and therapeutic value. Children should avoid products containing artificial sweeteners. Depending on the make-up of the drink, most of the commercial products are not recommended for nutritional or therapeutic use.

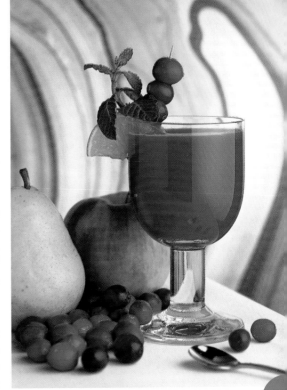

White refined sugar decreases both the nutritional and therapeutic value of cranberries. Use a bit of honey, maple syrup, natural fruit juices or molasses as substitutes.

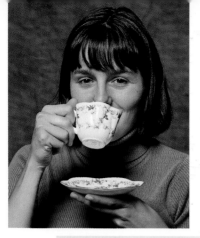

Cranberry Tea

Cranberry teas may contain artificial flavoring or other additives to make the product taste better. It is important to read the ingredients on the label before buying it if you intend to use it for its nutritional or therapeutic value.

Commercial Cranberry Juice

In 1994, J. Avron et al researched the reduction of bacteriuria (bacteria in the urine) and pyuria (pus in the urine) after the ingestion of cranberry juice and described it in the *Journal of the American Medical Association*. This double-blind study ran for six months and involved 153 women with an average age of 78.5 years who had similar medical problems, including pyuria and bacteriuria. They were divided into Group A and Group B. Group A drank a placebo that resembled cranberry juice in both taste and color while Group B drank cranberry juice. Group B tested positive for urinary tract infection only 42 percent as often as Group A. From this study, the researchers determined that real cranberry juice helps to reduce the number of white blood cells and the amount of bacteria found in the urine in this age group.

In 1968, Prodromas et al wrote in *Southwestern Medicine* of treating people with urinary tract infections with cranberry juice. Sixteen males and forty-four females, all with active urinary tract infections, took part in the study. Each drank 500 milliliters (16 ounces) of cranberry juice routinely. At the end of the study 73 percent had their urinary tract infections under control. After the study, 61 percent stopped drinking the juice and all had a recurrence of urinary infections.

In 1984 Sobota and Uro wrote in the *Journal of Urology* of their studies on the potential use of cranberry juice in treating urinary tract infections. Seventy-seven people took part in this study. All had been diagnosed with E. coli in their urine. Cranberry juice reduced the E. coli count by 75 percent or more in 60 percent of the participants.

A 1962 article in the *Wisconsin Journal of Medicine* described Meon's observation of the relief of symptoms in patients with chronic trigonitis and urethritis after they tried cranberries. A 66-year-old woman had taken various medications over a five-year period for chronic pyelonephritis (inflammation of the kidney and renal pelvis) with no relief. She began drinking 6 ounces of cranberry juice twice daily. After eight weeks the urine began to clear. This woman continued drinking the cranberry juice and after two and one-half years the urine was still free of infection.

Dried Cranberries

Dried cranberries really came into their own in the 1990s. Some nutrients will be lost during the heating and drying of the cranberries and a sweetener, often syrup, is added for taste. However, if the cranberry used is of good quality, dried cranberries make a relatively nutritious snack and are enjoyable to eat. Because of the amount of sugar in most of them, it is advisable to brush your teeth after eating them.

Therapeutic Forms of Cranberry · · · · ·

Scientific and traditional evidence indicates that the therapeutic effect of cranberries is greatest when they are in a form that is as close to their natural state as possible. Nonetheless, because of their exceptionally tart taste, short growing season and the difficulty of purchasing fresh cranberries year-round, few people are willing or able to consume therapeutic levels of the raw berries or natural juice. The drawbacks of cooked or sweetened cranberries have led to the development of various therapeutic cranberry products.

Liquid Concentrate

The product has been put into a condensed form by removing unwanted materials (often water), thus increasing its strength. There are various forms of concentrate available, such as concentrated cranberry juice.

Tincture

Tinctures are advantageous because they deliver a highly concentrated herbal substance in a small package. A few drops are sufficient for one dose. This type of remedy uses alcohol because it is a good solvent for extracting the most active components (the parts that are known to be beneficial); alcohol also serves as a stabilizer, preserving the tincture almost indefinitely. It has been proven that alcohol makes the walls of the stomach more permeable, which helps the body absorb the cranberry's qualities. For those who cannot have any alcohol at all, there is a new way of preparing tinctures, in a base of glycerine.

Extract

Extracts are herbal liquids prepared with either water or alcohol. Many herbs are now available in standardized extracts to assure their medicinal potency. This process of standardization is achieved by concentrating herbal extracts until their known active ingredients reach a specified level of potency. It is a way to combine science and nature for optimal advantage. However, many researchers and herbalists believe that you must consume the whole herb, as nature has provided it, to fully benefit from its therapeutic value. We cannot know for sure whether it is just certain components or the synergy of all parts of the herb that make it effective.

Capsules

Capsules may contain a certain amount of powdered crude herb, a powdered extract or a freeze-dried version of the cranberry (for more on freeze-dried cranberry capsules see the "Freeze-Drying" section on page 21). All packages of filled capsule shells should have the quantity of cranberry powder stated on the label, as well as a full disclosure of the ingredients. Capsule shells are generally made in one of two forms: gelatin and Vegicaps.

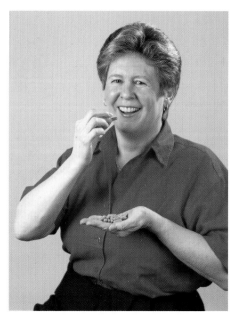

Tablets

To make tablets, the powdered herb is pressed into a solid form with a binding agent to help keep its shape. Depending on the tablet, it takes approximately thirty minutes to one hour to dissolve in the stomach. Some tablets can be difficult to digest for people with inadequate stomach acid production or insufficient digestive enzymes. One advantage to tablets is that since they are compressed under high pressure, often more ingredients can be contained in a single pill. However, tablets are not my favorite form of cranberry because they often contain many binders and excipients (fillers) and, as mentioned, digestion of tablets can be a problem.

Gelatin Capsule Shells

Most hard gelatin capsule shells are two parts, which are filled with a powder and then closed. They are one of the preferred therapeutic forms of cranberry for the following reasons:

- There is no product waste.
- They are in a controlled, condensed dosage.
- Dissolution of the capsule in a healthy person should occur within 30 minutes.
- They are easily opened to mix with food for people who have difficulty swallowing capsules.

Vegetarian Capsules

Some people object to gelatin capsules because gelatin is an animal-based product; Vegicaps are an excellent alternative. In my opinion they are the best way to take a therapeutic cranberry product for the following reasons:

- They are made from vegetable cellulose.
- The do not contain animal products and are therefore suitable for vegetarians.
- In a healthy stomach, Vegicaps dissolve within 20 minutes, making them perfect for people with low levels of stomach acid.
- There is no product waste.
- They provide a controlled, condensed dosage.
- They are easily opened to mix with food for people who have difficulty swallowing capsules.

Freeze-Drying

After doing much research, I believe a good freeze-dried product is the best way of receiving the therapeutic effect of cranberries. Freeze-drying preserves most of the fatty acids, volatile oils, polysaccharides, amino acids, enzymes, C and other vitamins, and various other nutrients. The more complete the end product, the greater the therapeutic value. Ordinary methods of preservation such as drying, home freezing, heating and alcohol or solvent extracting often alter or destroy important components.

Quality freeze-drying preserves the full range of ingredients, including color and taste, without subjecting the cranberries to heat or sweeteners.

Freeze-drying (lyophilization) as described by *Dorland's Illustrated Medical Dictionary* (28th edition) is "The creation of a stable preparation of a biological substance...by rapid freezing

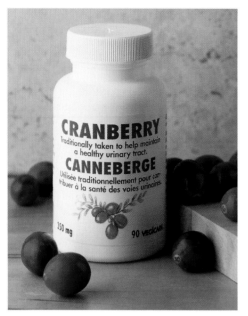

and dehydration of the frozen product under high vacuum." This method really developed during World War II, when it was used to preserve blood plasma. It has continued to be one of the most effective forms of preservation for more than fifty years.

The freeze-drying process: When done properly, the freeze-drying process occurs as follows: The freshly picked ripe cranberries are put into a deep freeze immediately, then dehydrated under very high vacuum. This removes virtually all the water and water vapor. This is done by converting the frozen cranberry from a solid to a vapor and then condensing it back to solid form again.

Once dehydration occurs the moisture content is usually less than 2 percent; this percentage is suitable to reduce the occurrence of reactions that degrade the product, to retard enzymatic activity and to completely prevent the growth of molds, yeast and micro-organisms. Since all cellular reactions require water to take place, and this product is virtually free of water, it is naturally preserved and will keep for years.

Francis Brinker, ND, wrote in the *Townsend Letters for Doctors* (Aug./Sept. 1989) how freeze-drying preserves the following:

- enzymes
- fatty acids
- amino acids
- proteins
- polysaccharides (many of these are important immune stimulants)
- volatile oils (these are particularly difficult to preserve using other techniques)
- physical properties
- chemical properties
- biological properties
- anthocyanidins

Growing evidence indicates that anthocyanidins from the

cranberry are very important and act on viruses, allergens and carcinogens and help fight night blindness and sore eyes.

After the freeze-drying process the product is encapsulated and bottled to protect it from the air. Some of the advantages of good-quality freeze-dried cranberry capsules include:
- no use of alcohol
- very little loss or degradation of potency
- chemical decomposition is minimized
- it is as close to fresh as possible
- no added sweeteners
- convenient and easy to carry when traveling
- no refrigeration required
- can be opened and the contents mixed with food
- long-term use has no detrimental effect, unlike the long-term use of antibiotics

Safety of Cranberries . . . .

Cranberries have been used as a well-tolerated, non-toxic and natural approach to treating urinary tract infections and related complications for centuries.

Long-Term Use with Antibiotics

In 1968, researchers Zinseer and Papas published their findings regarding cranberry juice in the treatment of urinary tract infections in *Southwestern Medicine*. These researchers spoke of the value of ingesting cranberry juice cocktail with an antibiotic. I know of a patient who had a chronic urinary tract infection and was on continual antibiotic therapy. When taking cranberry and an antibiotic together the infection finally cleared. He was then able to take the cranberry product successfully as a preventative without a return of the urinary tract infection. This person was taking a non-sweetened cranberry product, which no doubt had a lot to do with the excellent results. Extra sugar can lead to yeast infections in many people, particularly if the antibiotics are strong and the patient is taking them for a long time.

Allergies

Anyone can be allergic to anything, be it medication, flowers, paints, perfumes, food, etc. Very few people are allergic to cranberry. If you are able to eat cranberries in food forms, you most likely will be able to take it in other raw, natural states, provided there are no added fillers, preservatives or contaminants to which you may be allergic.

Interactions

After extensively researching both medical and traditional references, I have found no reported contraindications (unfavorable results when mixed with something else) for cranberry in any form; no negative interactions with any herbs, foods or drugs have been reported.

Cranberry for Additional Conditions . . . . .

The following are some of the reasons why these berries are so valuable in our everyday lives as food and for therapeutic purposes.

Ammonia Odors

Cranberries are noted for their excellent effect in preventing ammonia odors in urine. The compounds in cranberries are able to lower the pH of the urine to stop the degradation of the urine by E.coli, thus reducing the odor. In 1962 researcher Kraemer published in *Southwestern Medicine* his findings on cranberry juice and its value in the reduction of ammonia odors. He spoke of how cranberry juice acidifies the urine, preventing ammonia fermentation and gas production. A woman to whom I had suggested cranberry capsules wrote to me a while later and said, "I found while traveling long distances my urine had a very strong odor and became very cloudy. I wondered if I should ask my physician for an antibiotic for these times. I now take fresh freeze-dried cranberry capsules, as you suggested, twice daily when I am on a trip with very good results and, when at home, I take a capsule a day as a preventative—thank you."

There is a growing amount of modern scientific research indicating that certain bioflavonoids in cranberries...
- enhance the integrity and structure of the collagen matrix, thereby fighting osteoarthritis (joint disease); and
- help prevent and/or reverse macular degeneration, poor day and night vision, glaucoma and diabetic retinopathy.

The odor of ammonia in the urine is common among residents of nursing homes or hospitals, where many patients have bladder control problems. This includes mostly the elderly in long-term care facilities, but can include younger patients suffering from certain illnesses. Because this odor is strong and offensive, it is uncomfortable not only for the patients, but also for those around them.

The patients find the situation demoralizing and extremely uncomfortable, and often their buttocks develop small sores and within a short time, larger bed sores. Many of these people have indwelling catheters.

As Francis Brinker, ND, wrote in *Botanical Research Summaries*, 6 ounces of cranberry juice per day was of little help, but when subjects drank 16 ounces on a daily basis it generally reduced the pH level to 6.0 or less.

Bed Wetting

In *Secrets of the Chinese Herbalist*, author Richard Lucas describes the beneficial effects of cranberries in children troubled with bed wetting. One such testimonial reads as follows: "Our teenage

Cranberry juice provides beneficial effects for children troubled with bed wetting.

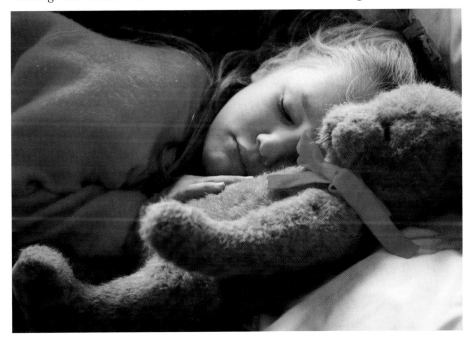

son wet the bed twice a night for the past two years. He had a kidney infection and passed cloudy, discolored urine. A small fortune was spent on medical treatments with little relief, so our family doctor finally advised that we take the boy to a specialist. Before the date of the appointment with the specialist, a friend told me that cranberry juice had cleared up her daughter's urinary infection and bedwetting problem.

"I bought a bottle of cranberry juice and gave my son 4 ounces about mid-afternoon. That night he didn't wet the bed. He has taken the juice daily for a year now and has slept dry every night except once. His kidney infection cleared up after he was on the juice for three weeks. The appointment with the specialist was never kept. Our family doctor checked my son and gave him a clean bill of health."

Candidiasis

Candida albicans is a common yeast found in everyone. Generally speaking this yeast lives in the gastrointestinal tract without causing any harm. If for some reason there is an overgrowth of it, it can lead to a serious disease called candidiasis. For more information on this disease read *Nature's Own Candida Cure*, by William G. Crook, MD (*alive* Health Guides, 2000). A physician should be consulted for proper diagnosis.

One patient I knew had a serious candidiasis condition and developed thrush. Thrush is an infection found in the mouth or throat, often caused by continual antibiotic therapy. This patient was told she would be on antibiotics for the rest of her life. Along with the antibiotics she began to take a freeze-dried cranberry product containing no added sugar and was able to go off the antibiotics (which helps her candidiasis). Subsequently the thrush infection has healed in her mouth. She now takes a freeze-dried cranberry product on a daily basis with excellent results.

Diabetes

Cranberries are safe for diabetics, who often suffer with kidney ailments, provided that the product is not accompanied by added sugar or harmful additives. Diabetics must remember that no matter how they are receiving their sugar—for example in fresh fruits and vegetables, milk, honey, white table sugar, brown sugar or preserved dishes—it is still a carbohydrate and eventually is broken down, ending up in the blood as a simple sugar. During my research I spoke with a registered dietician and she said 3 grams of dried or freeze-dried cranberry can easily be ingested on a daily basis with no effect on the blood sugar (providing the product is unsweetened).

Eye Disorders

There are many disorders of the eye; many are uncomfortable and very serious for the afflicted person, who may go through the trauma of losing most or all of their eyesight. It is important that we do whatever possible to keep the gift of vision, including using cranberries as a preventative. The following are some disorders of the eye and how cranberries can help.

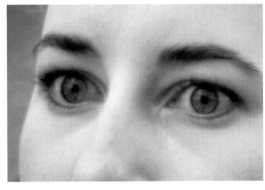

Macular degeneration: Macular degeneration is considered the number one cause of blindness in the elderly. This disorder occurs when a cyst-like lesion or sclerosis develops on the macula of the eye (located at the center of the retina and responsible for eye vision) and the person becomes either totally or partially blind. It can occur in anyone. Some forms of the condition are hereditary. It seems more prevalent in people over 55 or those who:

- have atherosclerosis (hardening of the arteries);
- have hypertension;
- have diabetic retinopathy;
- have been exposed to strong ultraviolet rays;
- live in areas with heavy pollution;
- smoke;
- eat a high-fat diet; or
- have sustained an injury to the eye.

Cranberries are rich in flavonoids. Flavonoids are believed to help in the treatment and prevention of this disorder, particularly in its early stages.

In 1997, Landrum et al at the Department of Chemistry at the Florida International University in Miami wrote in *Advances* in *Pharmacology* that the phytonutrient lutein was helpful in treating macular degeneration. Cranberries naturally contain lutein. Therefore, it would be an advantage for people with this illness to take cranberries in as close to their natural state as possible, thereby getting their full therapeutic value.

Night blindness: Night blindness does not mean that the sufferer is blind at night; rather, it means they have difficulty seeing well in dimming light.

Night blindness results when a person lacks rhodopsin. Rhodopsin is the purple portion of the eye necessary for night vision. The anthocyanins (a group of bioflavonoids) in cranberries appear to have the ability to treat night blindness because they stimulate the production of rhodopsin.

I have received excellent feedback from people taking cranberry, claiming improvement of this condition. One person wrote, "I decided cranberry capsules were worth a try as nothing else in the medical field had been of any help for my specific problem. This is a result of an injury to the eye as a small child, and the usual light sensitivity following cataract surgery. I have been both surprised and pleased with the results. I am able to withstand light to a much greater extent than before and if this discomfort should occur, it is of a much shorter duration. This is such an improved situation for me, I shall inform my ophthalmologist on my next visit."

Gout

The cause of gout is considered by many physicians to be both a metabolic and a renal (kidney) disorder. Therefore, the person often has a urinary tract infection. The renal disorder could be caused by a decrease in the renal clearance of uric acid (the person is unable to excrete sufficient uric acid) or the result of an overproduction of uric acid.

There is growing medical evidence that cranberries help lower uric acid levels in many people, because of the berry's bioflavonoid content. Along with other abilities, these compounds can prevent collagen destruction. Collagen is a protein that is the main component of connective tissue and its destruction is thought to promote inflammation. Since weight gain can be a problem for those with gout, a healthy diet and a cranberry product low in sugar are advisable, especially for people suffering from gout due to a renal disorder.

Incontinence

A national Angus Reid survey estimated that approximately 1.5 million ambulatory (walking) Canadians experience urinary incontinence. This survey did not include the approximately one million people in long-term care and similar facilities. The main reasons for incontinence are:

• urinary bladder infection (also called cystitis)
• urinary tract infection
• loss of bladder function

As we've already discussed, cranberry is very effective in preventing and clearing up these types of infections.

Multiple Sclerosis

Many people with multiple sclerosis are prone to urinary tract infections, especially if they require bladder catheterization frequently, or need a bladder catheter on a permanent basis (indwelling catheter). In either case, infections and ammonia odors are common. Often the person is on a long-term antibiotic and vitamin C regimen. The longer the person can stay off an antibiotic the better it is for them.

Cranberry is effective in clearing up the types of infections that lead to incontinence.

Cranberries contain both vitamin C and a substance that mimics the human Tamm-Horsfall glycoprotein, thus preventing E. coli bacteria from sticking to the walls of the urinary bladder. Cranberries help to clear the urinary tract infection as well as prevent urinary tract infections and ammonia odors for long periods of time in many people with this condition. In my opinion, cranberries need to be taken on the same daily basis as you would take medication if you wish to fight an infection or help to prevent one, in a situation such as this.

Premenstrual Syndrome

Along with other symptoms of premenstrual syndrome (PMS), many women have edema, or swelling, especially of the ankles and fingers, a bloated feeling in the abdomen and tender or swollen breasts. Cranberries have a mild diuretic effect and have helped many women with these symptoms.

Pregnancy

Pregnancy is a time when women are particularly prone to urinary tract infections. To date my extensive research has not shown any reasons why cranberries should be avoided during pregnancy. Many researchers feel that at least 1½ liters of cranberry juice must be consumed on a daily basis to provide a therapeutic effect.

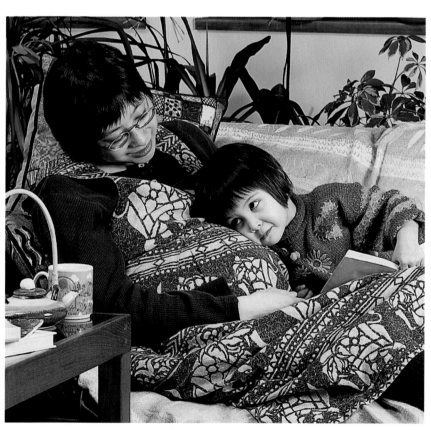

Diuretics

Cranberries have been traditionally known as having a mild diuretic effect for centuries. If you are using prescription diuretics, they should be taken at the time prescribed by your physician, which is generally in the morning. If there is any concern about taking both your prescription diuretic and cranberry, I would suggest taking cranberry after the noon meal or as otherwise directed by your physician.

Prostatitis

Prostatitis is an inflammation of the prostate gland, usually caused by bacteria from another part of the body (normally the urinary tract) invading it. The condition is very serious because, if left untreated, the inflammation can block the urine flow and urine retention could develop. If urine retention develops, the bladder will become distended, very tender and susceptible to infection. If the problem continues to be untreated, the kidneys can become infected.

With prostatitis, it is important for the body's bladder outlet (urethra) to be kept clear; otherwise, an obstruction could occur, resulting in uremia (a toxic condition in the blood that can result in death if not treated quickly).

Cranberries help fight urinary tract infection; therefore, they help to keep the bladder's outlet open. I am happy to say that many men are taking a good-quality cranberry product, to help control urinary tract infections, with excellent results.

Vaginal Infection

Most women will have a vaginal infection sometime during their lives. Normally bacteria and yeast live in the vagina in a balance that limits the growth of either one. However, if there is an excessive growth of one of them a vaginal infection can occur.

For most patients with vaginitis, a cranberry product can be very helpful since cranberries are acidic and help lower the pH level in the vaginal area. Yeast does not grow well in a low-pH or acidic environment.

Since increasing evidence seems to indicate that simple sugar helps feed yeast infections, women with this problem may be better off ingesting a cranberry product without added sugar.

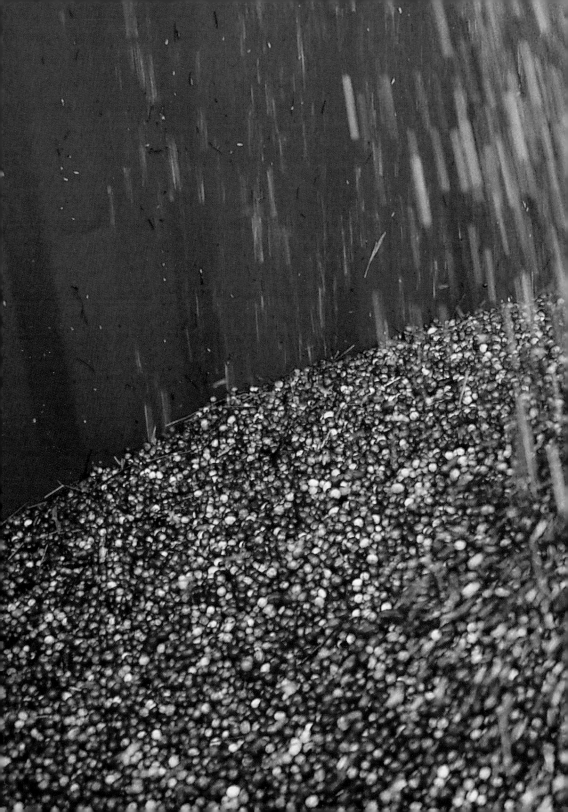

Cranberry Recipes

Why wait for Christmas or Thanksgiving to enjoy this wonderful berry? There are many ways to enjoy the taste and nutrition the cranberry provides.

Scrambled Eggs with Cranberry

Cranberries are the perfect food to complement a hearty, nutritional and cleansing breakfast.

3 red skin potatoes, cooked

2 tbsp cold-pressed olive oil

Sea salt or Herbamare to taste

1 tbsp parsley, chopped

2 tbsp natural, organic butter

2 large free-range eggs, beaten

2 tbsp cranberry preserve (page 40)

2 pieces whole grain toast

In a non-stick pan sauté potatoes in olive oil. Season potatoes with Herbamare vegetable salt or sea salt and pepper. Toss with half of the chopped parsley and set aside (covered) to keep warm.

In a non-stick sauté pan add butter, scramble the eggs and add remaining parsley. Season with Herbamare vegetable salt or sea salt and pepper. Serve with 2 tablespoons of cranberry preserve and toast.

Serves 2

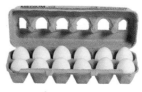

free-range eggs

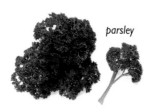

parsley

Cranberry Juice is Great!

See the Cranberry Juice recipe on page 38 and make it to complement this hearty breakfast. If you want a straight shot of cranberry nutrition leave out the apple and pear.

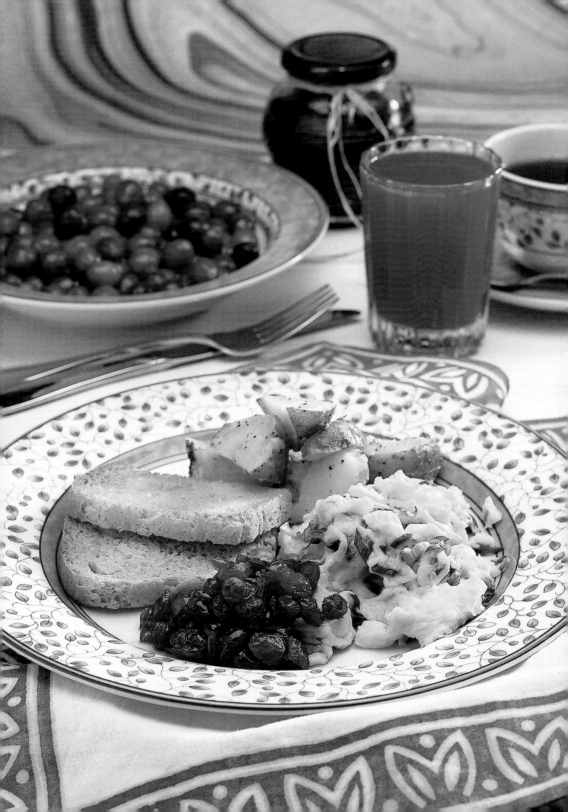

Waffles with Sun-Dried Cranberries

This tasty recipe is fun and versatile. It is perfect for afternoon tea or a child's birthday party and is always well received. You can also try the waffles with frozen cranberry yogurt (page 58).

1½ cups (350g) **whole wheat flour**

2 tsp **baking powder**

½ tsp **sea salt**

2 tsp **natural sugar cane crystals** (Sucanat or Rapadura)

2 **large free-range eggs, separated**

1 cup (240ml) **natural, organic milk**

⅓ cup (100ml) **butter, melted**

½ cup (120g) **sun-dried cranberries**

Natural, organic butter and maple syrup

Sift flour, baking powder and salt in a medium bowl. Stir in sugar cane crystals. In another bowl, combine egg yolks, milk and melted butter and beat well. Add to dry ingredients and beat thoroughly. In another bowl, beat egg white until stiff and fold into batter. Add sun-dried cranberries. Heat waffle iron, but do not grease. To test for correct heat, put 1 teaspoon of water inside waffle iron, close and heat. When steaming stops, heat is correct for cooking waffles. Spoon 1 tablespoon batter into center of each compartment. Close and cook until puffed and golden brown. Lift waffle out with a fork. Serve hot with butter and maple syrup, or cranberry butter (see recipe below).

Yields 6 waffles

Cranberry Butter

¼ cup (100g) **cranberry preserve** (page 40)

¼ lb (125g) **natural, organic butter** (room temperature)

½ tsp **lavender flowers** (optional)

Mix all ingredients together until smooth.

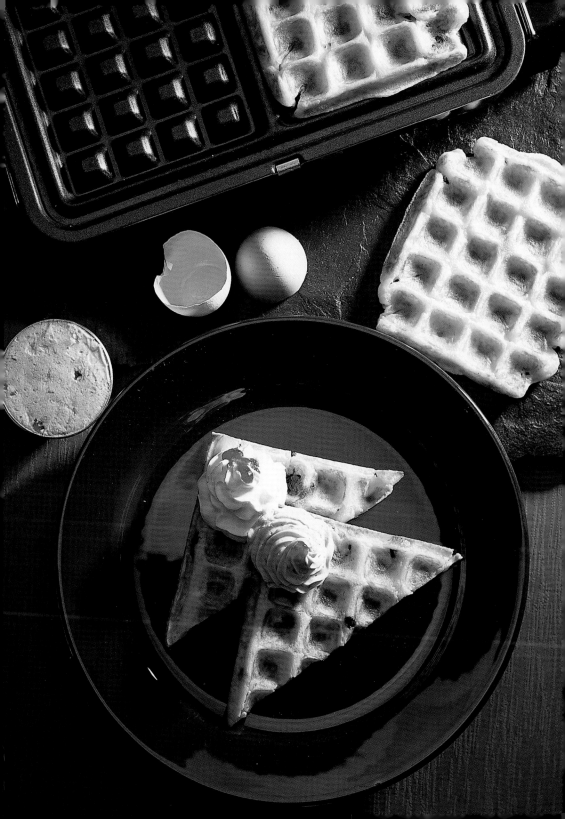

Cranberry-Apple-Pear Juice

Do you want some power in your juice? Well here it is! Let your imagination go wild and try cranberries with any kind of fruit you like for a custom power juice of your own. This combination tastes refreshing and provides a kick of energy.

2 lb (950g) fresh cranberries

1 large organic pear, cored

1 large organic apple, cored

2 tsp lemon or lime juice

2 tbsp honey

1 sprig fresh mint for garnish

Put cranberries, apple and pear through a juicer and mix the three juices. Pour into a glass and add lemon or lime juice and honey. Stir and garnish with fresh mint.

Serves 2

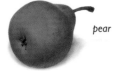

pear

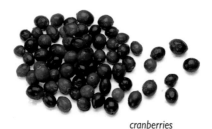

cranberries

If you don't have the pleasure of owning or using a juicer, simply add 1 cup (240ml) of water to the recipe and use a blender or food processor. Strain the pulp from the juice and enjoy!

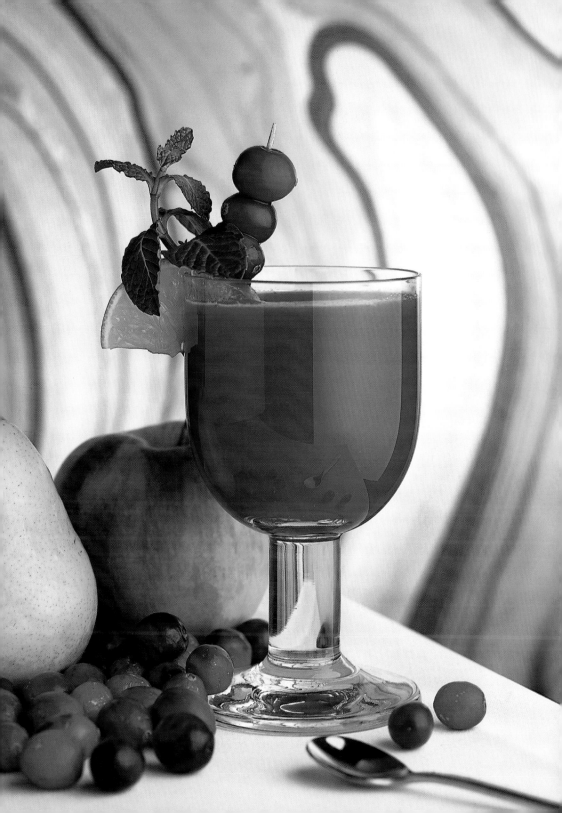

Cranberry Preserve

It isn't just for Christmas or Thanksgiving anymore. The delicious and healthful cranberry sauce adds a special and nutritious touch to any number of dishes. With some imagination, and a love for cranberries, you will come up with a lot of ideas!

4 cups (2lb) fresh cranberries

1 large organic orange, cut in ½" thick slices

1 large organic lemon, cut in ½" thick slices

1½ cups (350g) natural cane sugar crystals

2 cinnamon sticks

2 pieces star anise

1 piece cardamom

5 cloves

1 piece nutmeg

Pinch sea salt

½ q (½ l) water

Put all spices in cheesecloth and bundle into a little bag. (This makes it easier to remove the spices after cooking.) Put all ingredients in a large pot and slowly simmer on medium heat until all liquid is evaporated (approximately 20 to 30 minutes). Remove orange, lemon and the spice bag. You will see that the liquid has a jelly-like consistency. Set aside to cool. Once set keep covered and refrigerated.

lemon

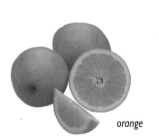

orange

Natural Sugar

Natural sugar crystals may be equally substituted for the white sugar called for in your recipes. There are many types of natural sugar crystals on the market. Some are superior to others simply because of the way they're made. I use either *Sucanat* or *Rapadura*. These natural sweeteners have a higher nutritional value than white sugar, with a natural rich flavor. Unlike white refined sugar, the process used to make these natural sugars preserves the natural taste and nutrition, without preservatives or additives, and actually has a lower level of sucrose.

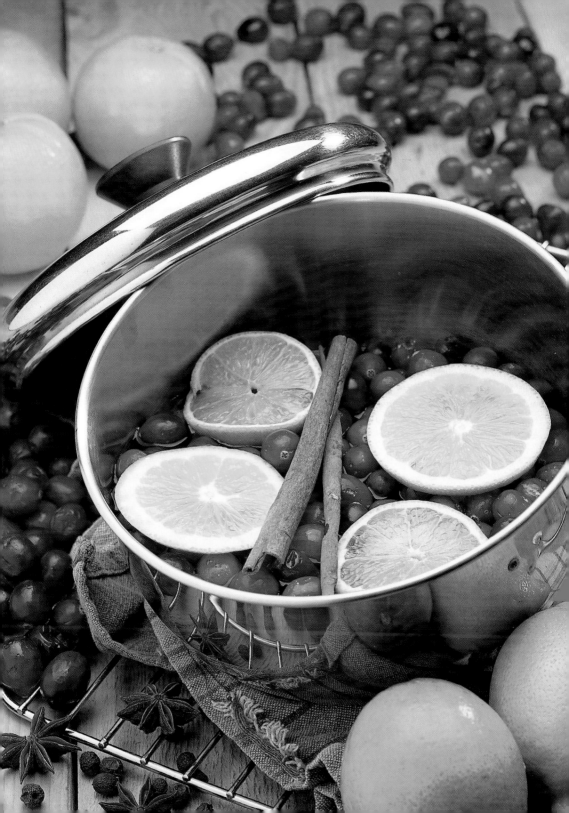

Marvelous Cranberry Muffins

Muffins are a treat and with this recipe, chalk full of cranberries, they are a nutritious treat! The entire family will enjoy them.

2 cups (500g) whole wheat flour

½ cup (150g) natural cane sugar crystals

5 tsp baking powder

½ tsp sea salt

¾ cup (300ml) natural, organic milk

⅓ cup (100ml) unprocessed coconut oil

I free-range egg, beaten

I cup (240g) sun-dried cranberries

¼ cup (100g) crumbled hazelnuts

I tbsp natural, organic butter

Heat oven to 400° F (200° C). Grease 12 muffin cups (bottom only) with butter or line with paper baking cups. In medium bowl, combine flour, sugar crystals, baking powder and sea salt; mix well. In another bowl combine milk, oil and egg. Add mixture to dry ingredients. Stir until dry ingredients are slightly moistened (batter will be lumpy). Add cranberries and hazelnuts; mix well.

Fill muffin cups ⅔ full. Bake for 20 to 25 minutes or until toothpick inserted in center comes out clean. Cool for 1 minute before removing from pan.

Yields 12 muffins

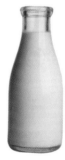

organic milk

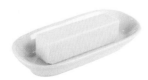

organic butter

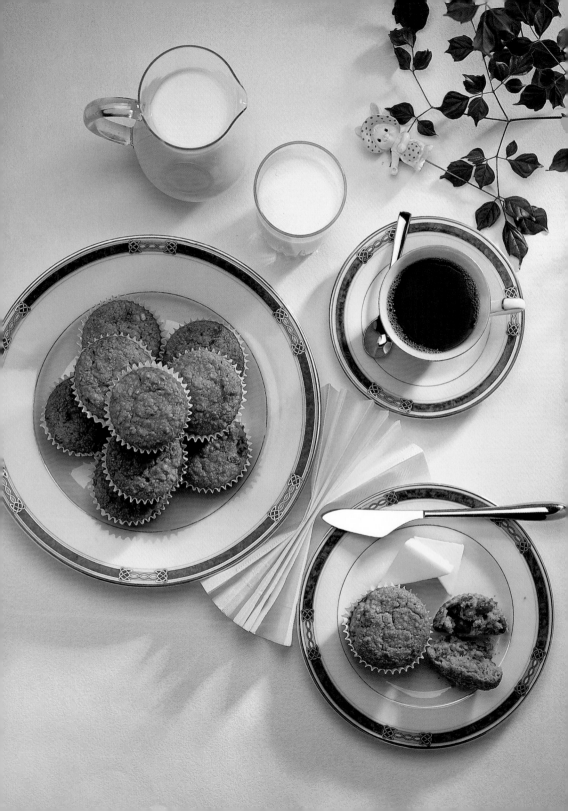

Vegetable Soup with Fresh Cranberries

This colorful, hearty soup is both delicious and energizing. Served hot on a cold day, it's a wonderful treat, full of vitamins, minerals and enzymes.

2 cloves garlic, minced

2 medium (200g) Yukon gold potatoes, cooked and cut in ½" cubes

1 cup (150g) carrot, cut in ½"cubes

1 cup (150g) celery, cut in ½"cubes

1 medium onion, chopped

½ cup (150g) red lentils, cooked

2 cups (500ml) vegetable broth

1 cup (150g) Brussels sprouts, quartered

2 large sage leaves

1 bay leaf

1 cup (200g) fresh cranberries

3 tbsp extra-virgin olive oil

Sea salt and pepper or Herbamare vegetable salt to taste

Sauté garlic and all vegetables (except Brussels sprouts and cranberries) in the olive oil. Add vegetable broth and simmer for 5 to 7 minutes. Add Brussels sprouts, all spices and fresh cranberries to the broth. Simmer for another 5 minutes. Add salt and pepper. If the taste is a little bit too tart for you add a teaspoon honey to the soup.
Serves 2

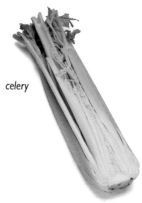
celery

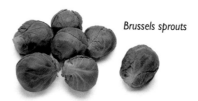
Brussels sprouts

Herbamare

This tasty natural seasoning is made with sea salt and 14 organic herbs. The special steeping process used to make this natural product allows the full herb and vegetable flavor to become concentrated in the salt crystal–preserving essential vitamins and minerals and providing ultimate zest.

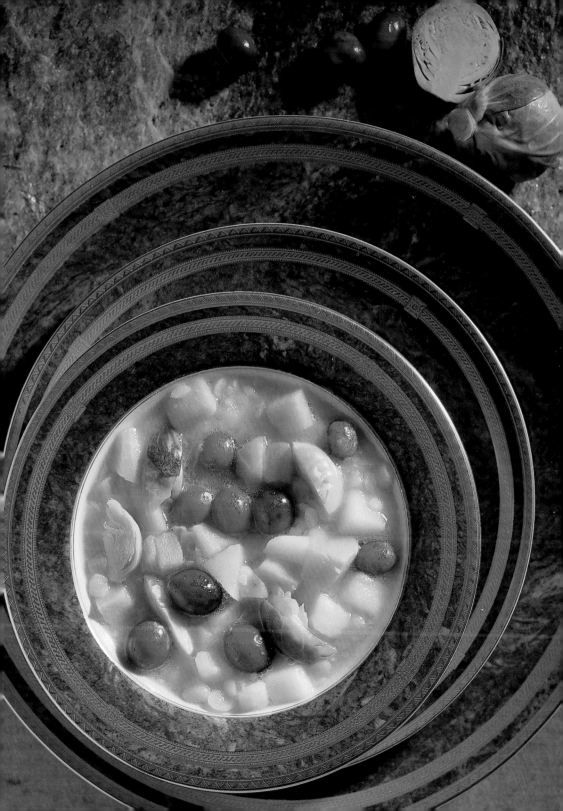

Chilled Cranberry-Papaya-Melon Soup

Wow! I cannot think of a better summer dish. You may call it an appetizer, a soup or dessert. Whatever you call it, people will love it. It's light, refreshing and very healthful.

Juice of 1 lb (500g) fresh cranberries, thoroughly strained

1½ tbsp maple syrup

1 tbsp lemon balm, finely chopped

Juice from ½ lemon or lime

Rind from ½ lime or lemon, finely chopped

1 cup (240g) papaya balls

1 cup (240g) honeydew melon balls

In a large bowl add maple syrup to cranberry juice. Then add lemon balm, juice and rind. Stir thoroughly before adding melon and papaya balls. Refrigerate for 20 minutes before serving. Garnish with more lemon balm or fresh mint.

Serves 2

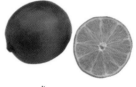

lime

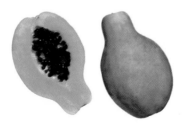

papaya

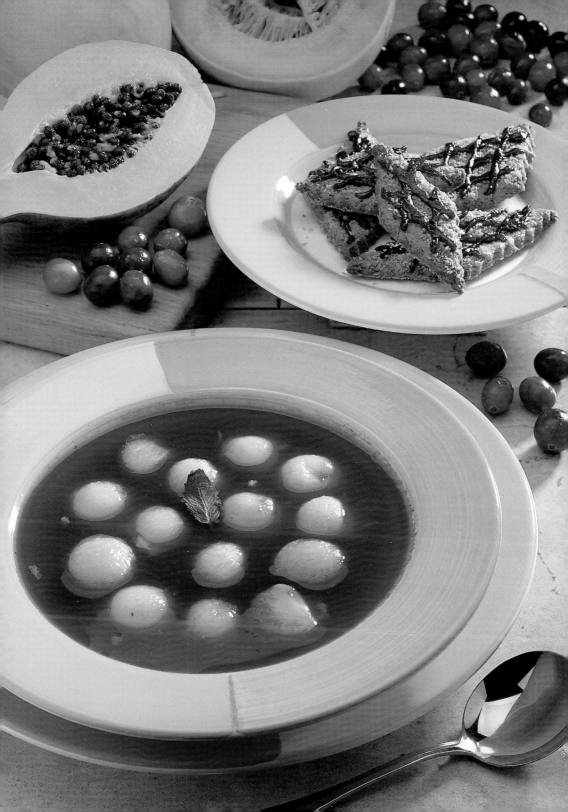

Salad with Pear and Cranberries

This is a healthy and delicious combination of fruit and salad. The sweetness of the fruit and the salty taste of the Gorgonzola cheese provide a unique flavor.

½ cup (120g) **sun-dried cranberries**

2 cups (150g) **fresh spinach leaves**

1 large **Belgian endive**

¼ cup (100g) **walnuts**

1 large **organic pear**

200 g **Gorgonzola cheese** (optional)

Separate the Belgian endive into individual leaves. Cut pear into segments. Toss endive and pear with spinach and sun-dried cranberries and then toss with mint-cranberry dressing (recipe below). Place in center of plate and add walnuts and Gorgonzola cheese.

Serves 2

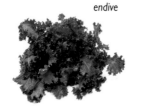

endive

Mint-Cranberry Dressing

2 tsp **cranberry sauce**

1 tsp **apple cider vinegar**

4 tbsp **olive oil**

1 sprig **mint, finely chopped**

Mix all ingredients together.

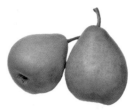

pear

Organic fruit and vegetables are becoming more and more readily available and are well worth the slightly higher price they cost. However, in the case where you cannot buy organic make sure you clean your produce carefully. An easy way to do this is with a non-toxic fruit and vegetable wash, which removes the residues of pesticides and chemical sprays. Look for a fruit and vegetable wash in your local health food store.

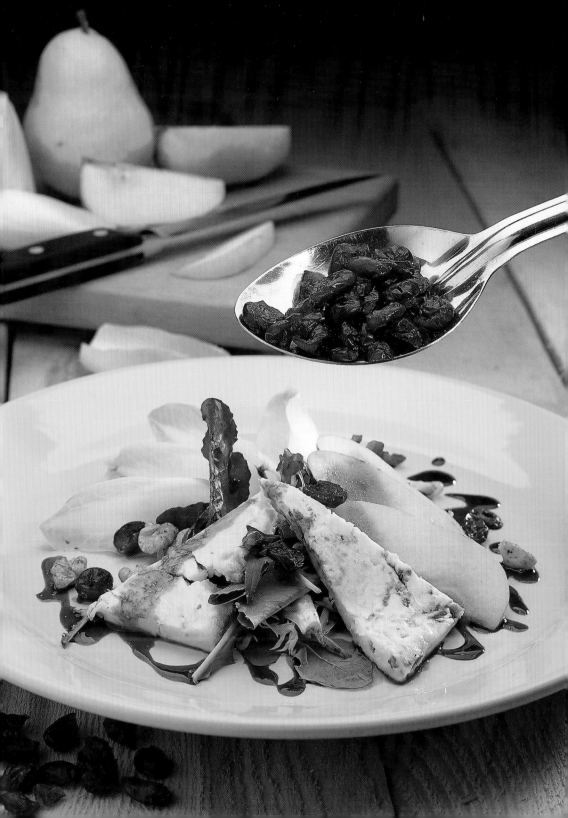

Cranberry Saffron Risotto

This original recipe features a little bit of Canada, a little bit of the Middle East and a little bit Italy! Saffron is considered to be the gold of the spices. It is not as cheap as most spices, but not as expensive as gold. Treat yourself and indulge in this wonderful taste. You will love it and so will your body as it is an extremely healthy combination!

½ cup (120g) **sun-dried cranberries**

I cup (230g) **risotto rice, uncooked**

I small onion, **finely chopped**

2 cloves garlic, minced

½ cup (150ml) **hot boiling water**

2½ cups (750ml) **vegetable broth**

½ tsp saffron

2 tbsp butter

2 tbsp extra-virgin olive oil

Sea salt and pepper to taste

In olive oil, sauté onion and garlic until translucent (not brown). Add risotto rice to the pot and continue to sauté for 2 to 3 minutes, then add vegetable broth. Stir slowly with a wooden spoon until the rice is loose and not lumpy. Add saffron to ½ cup of boiling water. Let it sit for at least 5 to 7 minutes until the water turns red (this is also called saffron tea, in kitchen terminology). After half of the rice liquid has evaporated add saffron tea and sun-dried cranberries. Stir until almost all liquid is evaporated and add the butter. Season with salt and pepper and mix all ingredients thoroughly.

Serves 2

If you like, substitute the saffron for paprika.

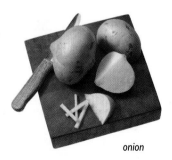

onion

Chopped orange rind gives a nice flavor to the risotto. Add about 1 tablespoon to the finished risotto.

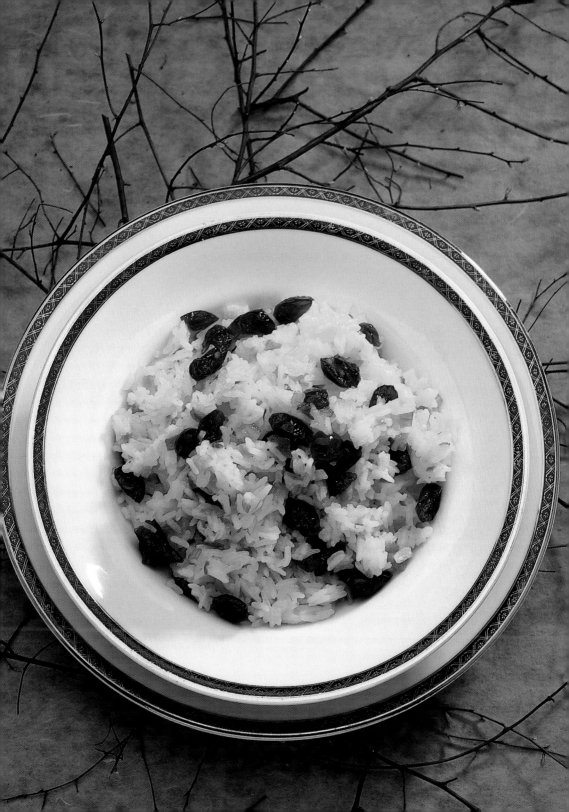

Spelt Spaghetti with Cranberries

Spelt is a relative of wheat and a hearty, tasty grain that is high in fiber. Combined with walnuts, mushrooms and cranberries, this pasta dish is simple to make, yet elegant to serve. It makes a complete meal with plenty of health benefits.

I cup (220g) fresh cranberries

3 cloves garlic, minced

I medium onion, chopped

¼ cup (125ml) organic vegetable broth

2 cups (300g) Portobello mushrooms, sliced

½ cup (150g) green onion, chopped

½ cup (200g) walnuts, halved

I tbsp dill, chopped

I tbsp natural, organic butter

250 g spelt spaghetti, cooked al dente

3 tbsp extra-virgin olive oil

Sea salt and pepper or Herbamare to taste

Sauté garlic and onion in olive oil until translucent. Add mushrooms and sauté for another 2 minutes. Add cranberries, vegetable broth and all other ingredients. Mix thoroughly and add cooked pasta. Toss very well.

Serves 2

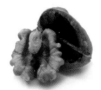

walnut

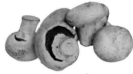

mushroom

To correctly clean your mushrooms use either a dry kitchen cloth or a pastry brush. Just brush the dirt off the mushroom. Or, you can carefully peel the top skin of the mushroom with a paring knife. Do not clean your mushrooms with water. Their spongy consistency absorbs the water (and dirt), and the water also encourages them to oxidize and turn brown.

"Al dente" is Italian and means cooked but still firm to the bite.

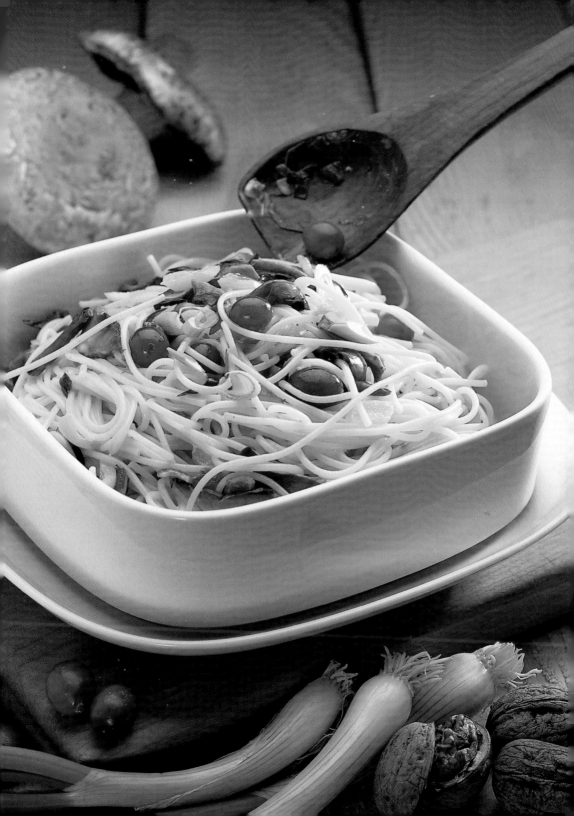

Cranberry-Polenta with Sautéed Vegetables

This creative, yet easy to make, recipe makes wonderful use of the North American cranberry in a traditional Italian dish. The combination is as nutritious as it is tasty.

Sautéed Vegetables:

1 medium zucchini, cut in ½" slices

1 medium eggplant, cut in ½" slices

1 Belgium endive, cut in half

1 yellow bell pepper, cut lengthwise in 4" pieces

1 red bell pepper, cut lengthwise in 4" pieces

2 baby carrots

1 oz (30ml) cranberry preserve (page 40)

3 tbsp extra-virgin olive oil

Herbamare vegetable salt to taste

Polenta:

½ cup (120g) sun-dried cranberries

1 cup (240g) corn meal or Polenta flour

¼ cup (80) green onion, finely chopped

2 small shallots, minced

1 tsp garlic, minced

1 tbsp thyme leafs

1 tbsp natural, organic butter

2¼ cup (480ml) water

2 tbsp extra virgin olive oil

Sea salt and pepper to taste

Vegetables: Pre-heat oven to 380° F (190° C). Brush all vegetables with olive oil, place them on a cookie sheet and put them in the oven for about 10 minutes until golden brown on both sides. Season with salt and pepper or alternatively Herbamare vegetable salt.

Polenta: In a saucepan, sauté onion and garlic until transluscent. Add water and all other ingredients except Polenta flour. Slowly, while stirring, add Polenta flour and keep stirring until the combination becomes thick and smooth. Grease a small round cake form dish with butter and pour the Polenta mixture into the form where it will cool and set. Before serving, cut into pieces and heat it at 330° F (160° C) for 5 minutes.

Serve with cranberry preserve (page 40).

Serves 2

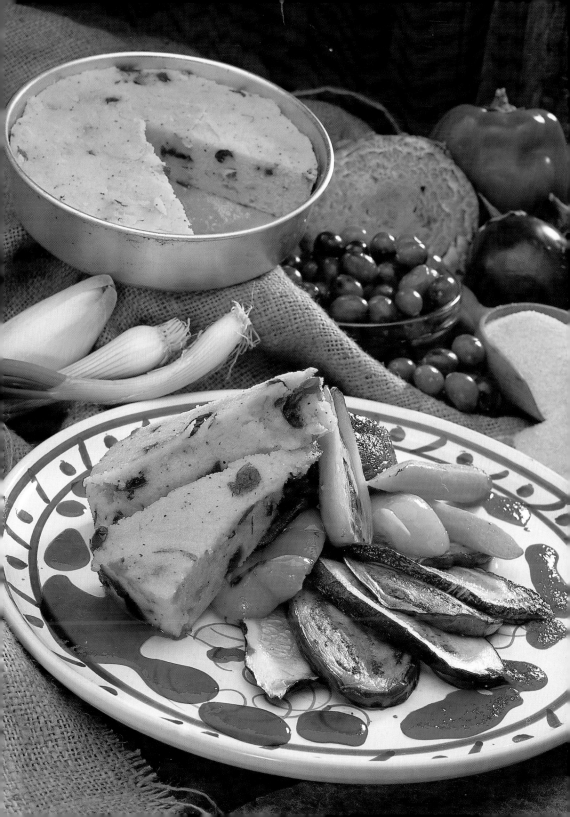

Cranberry Sorbet

This recipe offers a sweet and delicious way to seduce your guests with cranberries. Sorbet often is served between two courses to stimulate the appetite, or it makes a wonderful dessert, of course.

1 cup (250ml) **fresh cranberry juice**

½ cup (125ml) **water**

1 tsp **freshly squeezed lemon juice**

1 tsp **lemon rind, finely chopped**

1 tsp **fresh mint, finely chopped**

¼ cup (80g) **natural cane crystals**

¼ cup (80ml) **honey**

1 **egg white**

Mix all ingredients together, except for the egg white. Beat egg white until stiff and fold into mixture. Pour mixture into ice cube trays. Freeze for 4 to 5 hours, or until firm.

Serves 2

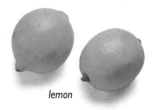

lemon

Frozen Cranberry Yogurt

1 cup (250g) **cranberry preserve** (page 40)

2 cups (500g) **organic plain yogurt**

½ cup (125ml) **natural whipping cream**

1 tbsp **honey**

¼ cup (60g) **sun-dried cranberries**

Place all ingredients into a food processor and set on pulse speed for 1 to 2 minutes, or beat on high with an electric hand mixer, until consistency is smooth. Pour into ice cube trays or a square cake form (you could also use a plastic container). Freeze for 6 hours or longer.

Serves 2

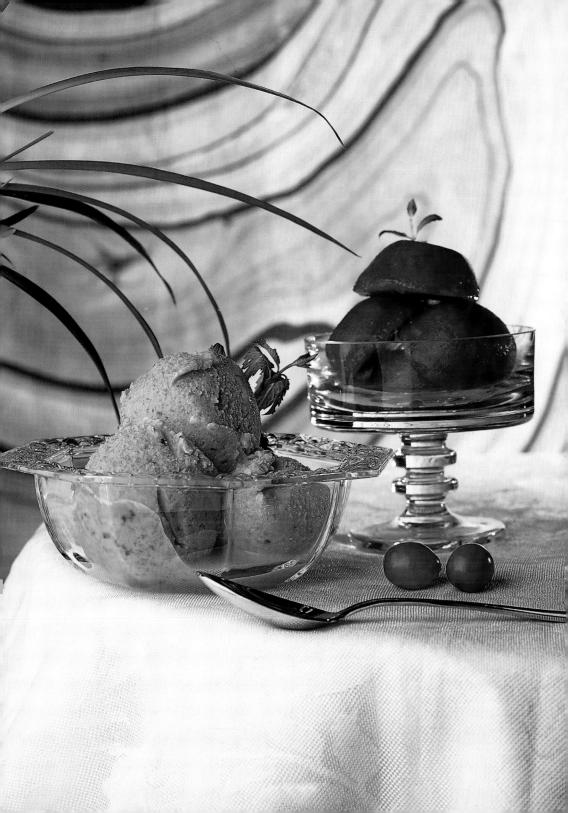

Cranberry Flaky Cookies

These cookies make a nice and healthy Christmas treat, but they're also great to make and share year round.

2 cups (350g) **whole wheat flour**

2 tbsp gluten flour

2 tsp baking powder

⅔ cup (200g) **natural cane crystals**

½ tsp sea salt

⅔ cup (200g) **grated hazel nuts** (plus 2 extra tbsp for garnish)

1 tsp almond extract

1 tsp natural vanilla extract

5 tbsp cold water

½ cup (125g) **natural, organic butter**

1 egg, beaten

1 cup (240g) **Cranberry Preserve** (page 40)

butter (to grease parchment paper)

parchment paper for cookie sheet

Combine flour, baking powder, cane crystals, salt and hazelnuts in a bowl and mix thoroughly. Mix the almond extract, vanilla extract and water together and add to dry ingredients. Add ½ cup of butter, work into dough and let it rest in the refrigerator for 1 hour. Once removed from refrigerator, form small balls and set them on butter-greased parchment paper. Press cookie balls down slightly with the palm of your hand then, with your thumb, put a small indent in the middle of each cookie.

Bake it in a pre-heated oven at 350° to 400° F (175° to 200° C) for 20 minutes. Half way through the baking time brush the cookies with the beaten egg and sprinkle the rest of the hazelnuts on top, then continue baking. Remove from the oven and immediately dot the cranberry preserve into the indent of each cookie.

Yields 1 dozen cookies

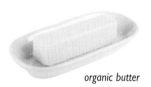

organic butter

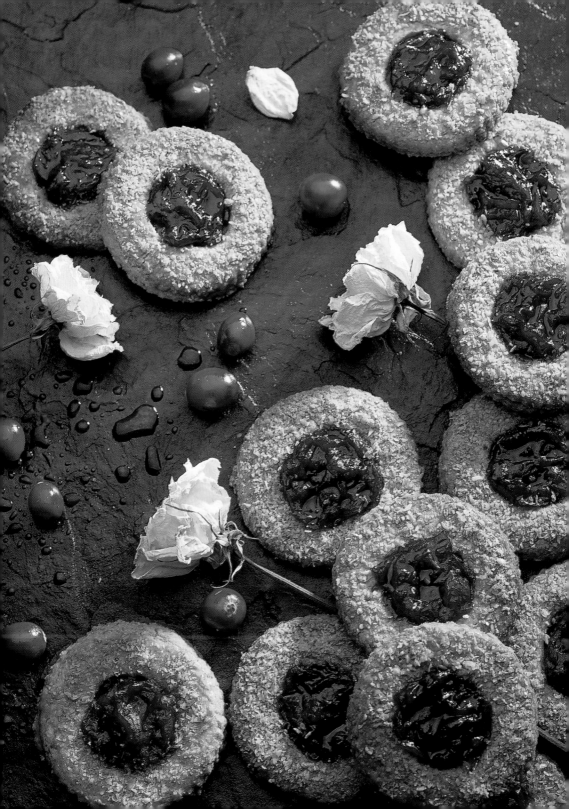

Cranberry Cake

½ **lb** (240g) **cranberries**

2 **tbsp brown rum** (or black Jasmin tea)

2 **tbsp water**

1 **tbsp maple syrup**

1 **tsp orange rind**

1 **tsp lemon rind**

3 **free-range eggs**

½ **cup** (120g) **natural cane crystals**

1 **vanilla bean or 2 tsp natural vanilla extract**

⅛ **tsp sea salt**

½ **cup** (120g) **spelt flour or whole wheat flour**

⅛ **cup** (50ml) **milk**

1 **tsp hazelnut or walnut oil**

Pinch nutmeg

Natural organic butter

Gently warm cranberries with rum, water, maple syrup, orange rind and lemon rind until cranberries get slightly soft. Set aside.

Beat eggs with natural cane crystals. Cut the vanilla bean lengthwise and scrape the seeds out. Add vanilla seeds to the mixture. Add salt and flour and slowly add milk. With a whisk, carefully mix together then add oil and nutmeg. Add cranberries to mixture, but do not stir.

Grease the cake form with the butter and pour the mixture into the cake form. Preheat oven to 350° F (180° C) and bake for 40 to 45 minutes on the lower shelf of your oven. Serve warm.

Serves 4 to 6

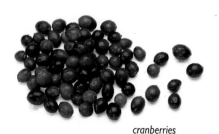

cranberries

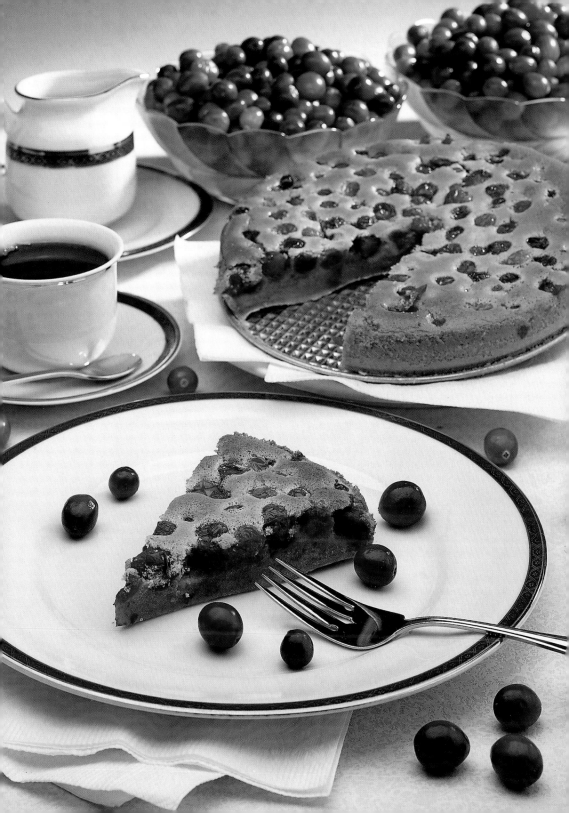

references

Ancharski, Michael, ND. "Fresh Freeze-Dried Botanical Medicine." Complementary Medicine. (July/Aug. 1986).

Avron, J. et al. "Reduction of Bacteriuria and Pyuria After Ingestion of Cranberry Juice." Journal of the American Medical Association. 271 (1994): 751.

Barney, Paul. The Journal of the American Botanical Council and the Herb Research Foundation. 38 (winter 1998).

Blake, Steven. Global Herb Data Base. (1994).

Blatherwick. "The Specific Role of Foods in Relation to the Composition of Urine." Archives of Internal Medicine. 14 (1914): 409.

—— and M.I. Long. "Studies of Urinary Acidity: The Increased Acidity Produced by Eating Prunes and Cranberries." Journal of Biological Chemistry. 57 (1923): 81518.

Brinker, Francis. Botanical Research Summary. Sandy, OR: Eclectic Medical Publications.

——. "Lyophilization of Fresh Medicinal Plants." Townsend Letter for Doctors. (Aug./Sept. 1989).

Dorland's Illustrated Medical Dictionary, 28th ed. Philadelphia: W.B. Saunders Co., 1998.

Dulawa, J.k. et al. "Tamm-Horsfall Glycoprotein Interferes with Bacterial Adherence to Human Kidney Cells." European Journal of Clinical Investigation. 18 (1988): 8791. "Cranberry Juice Inhibits Bacterial Adherence." Vol. 33 (1989).

Eden, C.S. et al. "Adhesion of Escherichia Coli to Human Uroepithelial Cells in Vitro." Infection and Immunity. Vol. 18, no. 3 (Dec. 1977): 76774.

Gursche, Siegfried, et al. Encyclopedia of Natural Healing. Vancouver: Alive Books, 1997.

Fellers, C.R. et al. "Effect of Cranberries on Urinary Acidity and Blood Alkali Reserve." Journal of Nutrition. 7 (1933): 455.

"Food Bites-Study Backs Cranberry Juice." The Washington Post. (Feb. 15, 1994, final edition).

Kahn, D.H. et al. "Effect of Cranberry Juice on Urine." Journal of the American Dietetic Association. 51 (1967): 251.

Konowalchuk, J. and J. Spiers. "Anti-viral Effect of Commercial Juices and Beverages." Applied Envir. Microbiology. 35 (1978): 1219.

Kraemer, R.J. "Cranberry Juice and the Reduction of Ammoniacal Odor of Urine." Southwestern Medicine. 45 (1962): 211.

Landrum, John T. et al. "Macular Degeneration." Advances in Pharmacology. (1997).

Lawrence, H.E. Review of Natural Products. (July 1994).

Lucas, Richard. Secrets of the Chinese Herbalists, Vol. 1: Chinese Herb Remedies for Urinary Disorders. Parker Publishing Co., 1987.

Meon, D.V. "Observations of the Effectiveness of Cranberry Juice in Urinary Infections." Wisconsin Journal of Medicine. 61 (1962): 282.

Neilsen, F.H. "Boron-An Overlooked Element of Potential Nutrition Importance." Nutrition Today. (Jan./Feb. 1988): 47.

Ofek, Itzhak et al. "Anti-Escherichia Coli Adhesion Activity of Cranberry and Blueberry Juices." New England Journal of Medicine. Vol. 324, no. 22 (May 30, 1991): 1599.

Papas, P.N. et al. "Cranberry Juice in the Treatment of Urinary Tract Infections." Southwestern Medicine. 47 (1966): 17.

Prodromos, P.N. et al. "Cranberry Juice in the Treatment of Urinary Tract Infection." Southwestern Medicine. 47 (1968): 17.

Quick, A.J. "Conjugation of Benzoic Acid in Man." Journal of Biological Chemistry. 92 (1931): 65.

Roger, June. "Pass the Cranberry Juice." Nursing Times. Vol. 87, no. 48 (November 27, 1991).

Schmidt, R.D. and Sobota, A.E. "An Examination of the Anti-adherence Activity of Cranberry Juice on Urinary and Non-urinary Bacterial Isolates." Microbial. 55 (1988): 173181.

Sobota, A.E. and J. Uro. "Inhibition of Bacterial

Adherence by Cranberry Juice: Potential Use for the Treatment of Urinary Tract Infection." Journal of Urology. Vol. 131, no. 5 (May 1984): 101316.

Thom, J. et al. "The Influence of Refined Carbohydrates on Urinary Calcium Secretion." British Journal of Urology. 50 (1978): 93102.

Uehling, David T. "What Makes Bacteria Stick to the Bladder Mucosa." Journal of Urology. 140 (July 1988): 156.

Walsh, B. "Urostomy and Urinary pH." Journal J et Nursing. Vol. 19, no. 4 (July/Aug. 1992): 11013.

Wightman, J.D. and T.E. Wrolated. "Anthocyanin Analysis as a Measure of Glycosidase Activity in Enzymes for Juice Processing." Journal of Food Science. Vol. 60, no. 4 (July/Aug 1995): 86267.

Zinseer, H.H. et al. "Management of Infected Stones with Acidifying Agents," New York State Journal of Medicine. 68 (1968): 3001.

Zinseer, H.H. "Newer Antibacterial Drugs in Urological Infections." Medical Clinics of North America. 48 (1964): 293.

sources

for freeze-dried cranberry:
CRAN-DALE INC.
423 Booth Drive
Winnipeg, Manitoba
R3J 3M9
Tel: (204) 837-1594
Fax: (204) 837-6074
E-mail: cran_dale@hotmail.com

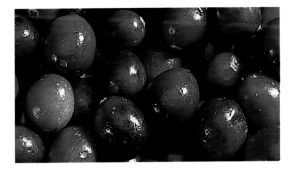

First published in 2000 by
alive books
7436 Fraser Park Drive
Burnaby BC V5J 5B9
(604) 435–1919
1-800–661–0303

© 2000 by **alive** books

Artwork:
    Liza Novecoski
    Terence Yeung
    Raymond Cheung
Food Styling/Recipe Development:
    Fred Edrissi
Photography:
    Edmond Fong
Photo Editing:
    Sabine Edrissi-Bredenbrock
Editing:
    Sandra Tonn
    Donna Dawson

Canadian Cataloguing in
Publication Data

Dales, Phyllis I. and Dales, Bruce
    Cranberry

(**alive** natural health guides, 10
ISSN 1490-6503)
ISBN 1-55312-007-8

Printed in Canada

Revolutionary Health Books

alive Natural Health Guides

Each 64-page book focuses on a single subject, is written in easy-to-understand language and is lavishly illustrated with full color photographs.

New titles will be published every month in each of the four series.

Self Help Guides

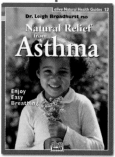

alive Natural Health Guides 12
Dr. Leigh Broadhurst PhD
Natural Relief from Asthma
Enjoy Easy Breathing

other titles to follow:

- **Nature's Own Candida Cure**
- **Natural Treatment for Chronic Fatigue Syndrome**
- **Fibromyalgia Be Gone!**
- **Heart Disease: Save Your Heart Naturally**

Healthy Recipes

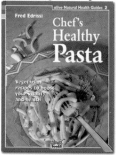

alive Natural Health Guides 2
Fred Edrissi
Chef's Healthy Pasta
Vegetarian recipes to boost your vitality and health

other titles to follow:

- **Baking with the Bread Machine**
- **Baking Bread: Delicious, Quick and Easy**
- **Healthy Breakfasts**
- **Desserts**
- **Smoothies and Other Healthy Drinks**

Healing Foods & Herbs

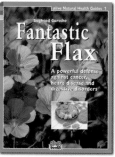

alive Natural Health Guides 1
Siegfried Gursche
Fantastic Flax
A powerful defense against cancer, heart disease and digestive disorders

other titles to follow:

- **Calendula: The Healthy Skin Helper**
- **Ginkgo Biloba: The Good Memory Herb**
- **Rhubarb and the Heart**
- **Saw Palmetto: The Key to Prostate Health**
- **St. John's Wort: Sunshine for Your Soul**

Lifestyle & Alternative Treatments

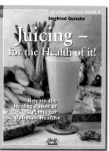

alive Natural Health Guides 3
Siegfried Gursche
Juicing – for the Health of it!
Release the Healing Power of Plants for Optimum Health

other titles to follow:

- **Maintain Health with Acupuncture**
- **The Complete Natural Cosmetics Book**
- **Kneipp Hydrotherapy at Home**
- **Magnetic Therapy and Natural Healing**
- **Sauna: Your Way to Better Health**

alive books
Vancouver
Canada

Great gifts at an amazingly affordable price **$9.95 Cdn / $8.95 US / £8.95 UK**

alive Natural Health Guides are available in health and nutrition centers and in bookstores. For information or to place orders please dial 1-800-663-6513